Snoring facts and challenges

Anti-snoring facts and tricks to stop snoring when asleep. (night)

Brad Attwood

Table of content

Chapter1:Introduction to Sleep

Sleep is an essential biological process that plays a vital role in our overall health and well-being. It is a natural and recurring state of reduced consciousness and decreased responsiveness to the external environment. While we may often think of sleep as a passive state, it is a dynamic process during which our bodies undergo numerous complex physiological and psychological changes.

Humans spend approximately one-third of their lives sleeping, and the quality and quantity of sleep have a profound impact on our physical health, mental function, and emotional well-being. However, despite its importance, sleep is often undervalued and neglected in today's fast-paced society.

The sleep-wake cycle, also known as the circadian rhythm, regulates our sleep patterns.

This internal clock is influenced by external cues such as light and darkness, which help synchronize our sleep-wake cycle with the natural 24-hour day. Disruptions to this cycle, such as shift work or jet lag, can lead to difficulties in falling asleep or staying asleep, resulting in sleep disorders.

During sleep, the body goes through different stages that are characterized by distinct patterns of brain activity.

These stages include non-rapid eye movement (NREM) sleep and rapid eye movement (REM) sleep. NREM sleep can be further divided into three stages: N1, N2, and N3. Each stage serves a specific function in maintaining our overall health.

Sleep plays a crucial role in physical restoration and healing. It is during sleep that the body repairs and rejuvenates itself.

Growth hormone is released, promoting tissue repair, muscle growth, and bone strength. Sleep also supports a healthy immune system, as it allows the body to produce and release cytokines, which aid in fighting off infections and inflammation.

Furthermore, sleep is closely intertwined with cognitive function and memory consolidation. Research has shown that sleep enhances learning, memory formation, and problem-solving abilities.

It is during sleep that the brain processes and consolidates information gathered throughout the day, leading to improved performance and mental agility.

Lack of sufficient sleep or poor sleep quality can have significant consequences on our health and daily functioning. Sleep deprivation has been linked to a wide range of physical and mental health problems, including obesity, diabetes, cardiovascular disease, impaired immune function, depression, anxiety, and decreased cognitive performance.

In today's modern society, various factors contribute to the prevalence of sleep problems. Hectic lifestyles, excessive screen time, demanding work schedules, and stress are just a few examples. It is crucial, however, to prioritize sleep and adopt healthy sleep habits to maintain optimal well-being.

Creating a conducive sleep environment and practicing good sleep hygiene can greatly improve the quality and quantity of sleep.

This includes establishing a regular sleep schedule, ensuring a comfortable and quiet sleeping environment, avoiding stimulants like caffeine and electronic devices close to bedtime, and engaging in relaxation techniques before sleep.

In conclusion, sleep is a fundamental biological process that is vital for our physical health, mental well-being, and overall quality of life.

Understanding the importance of sleep and adopting healthy sleep practices can significantly enhance our daily functioning, cognitive abilities, and overall sense of well-being. By valuing and prioritizing sleep, we can unlock the numerous benefits it offers and lead healthier, happier lives.

Types of sleeping and when to have them

In this article, we will explore different types of sleep and discuss the optimal times to have them for a healthy sleep routine.

Nighttime Sleep:
Nighttime sleep, also known as nocturnal sleep, is the most common type of sleep. It occurs during the nighttime hours when the body's internal clock, known as the circadian rhythm, signals the brain to release sleep-inducing hormones.

The optimal duration for nighttime sleep varies among individuals, but most adults require around 7-9 hours of uninterrupted sleep each night.

Napping:
Napping is a short period of sleep taken during the day to alleviate sleepiness and enhance alertness. There are several types of naps, each serving different purposes:

Power Nap: A power nap typically lasts for 10-20 minutes and aims to boost alertness and productivity. It helps combat drowsiness and improves cognitive function without causing grogginess upon awakening.

Short Nap: A short nap lasts between 20-30 minutes and provides similar benefits to a power nap. It enhances alertness, creativity, and memory consolidation, making it ideal for individuals seeking a quick energy boost.

Long Nap: A long nap, lasting 60-90 minutes, involves a complete sleep cycle. It allows for both non-rapid eye movement (NREM) and rapid eye movement (REM) sleep stages. Long naps promote memory formation, creativity, and emotional processing, but they may lead to sleep inertia upon awakening.

Recovery Sleep:
Recovery sleep refers to an extended period of sleep that helps individuals compensate for lost sleep or manage sleep debt.

It is particularly beneficial for those who have experienced sleep deprivation due to a hectic schedule, illness, or other factors. Recovery sleep often involves sleeping longer than usual, allowing the body to restore its energy levels and promote physical and mental recovery.

Split Sleep:

Split sleep is a sleep pattern that involves dividing the sleep period into two separate segments. Instead of sleeping for a continuous block of time, individuals have two sleep periods separated by a period of wakefulness. This sleep pattern was common in preindustrial societies and is still practiced in certain cultures. Some people may naturally prefer a split sleep pattern, while others adopt it due to work schedules or personal preferences.

Shift Work Sleep:

Shift work sleep refers to sleep patterns adapted by individuals who work during non-traditional hours, such as overnight or rotating shifts. Shift workers often face challenges in maintaining a regular sleep routine due to disrupted circadian rhythms. They may experience sleep disturbances, excessive daytime sleepiness, and an increased risk of chronic health conditions. To optimize their sleep, shift workers can create a conducive sleep environment, practice good sleep hygiene, and establish consistent sleep and wake times.

Conclusion:
Understanding the different types of sleep and their optimal times can help individuals establish a healthy sleep routine. Nighttime sleep serves as the foundation for restorative rest while napping can provide quick bursts of energy and alertness throughout the day. Recovery sleep allows individuals to replenish lost sleep, while split sleep and shift work sleep patterns cater to unique lifestyles and work schedules. By prioritizing sleep and adopting appropriate sleep patterns, individuals can optimize their overall well-being and lead more productive lives.

Chapter2:What is snoring

Cause of snoring

Snoring: Causes, Effects, and Treatment Options

What is snoring

Snoring is a common sleep disorder characterized by the production of loud and harsh sounds during sleep. It occurs when there is an obstruction to the normal flow of air through the air passages in the nose and throat. This obstruction causes the soft tissues in the throat, such as the tongue, to vibrate, resulting in the sound of snoring.

Snoring can be caused by a variety of factors, including age, gender, obesity, alcohol consumption, smoking, allergies, and sleep position. It can also be a symptom of an underlying medical condition such as sleep apnea.

Snoring can be disruptive to both the snorer and their partner, leading to disturbed sleep, daytime fatigue, and other health problems. It can also cause social embarrassment and strain on relationships.

There are various treatments available for snoring, including lifestyle changes, such as weight loss and smoking cessation, positional therapy, nasal sprays, and oral devices that help to keep the airways open. In some cases, surgery may be required to correct the underlying issue causing the snoring.

If you or someone you know snores regularly and experiences symptoms such as daytime fatigue, morning headaches, or pauses in breathing during sleep, it is important to seek medical attention to determine the underlying cause and receive appropriate treatment.

Snoring: Causes, Effects, and Treatment Options

Snoring is a common sleep disorder that affects millions of people worldwide. It is characterized by the production of loud and harsh sounds during sleep, caused by the obstruction of airflow through the air passages in the nose and throat. While it may seem like a minor annoyance, snoring can have significant effects on both the snorer and their sleeping partner. In this article, we will explore the causes of snoring, its effects on sleep and health, and the various treatment options available.

Causes of Snoring:

Snoring can have multiple causes, and understanding them is crucial in determining the most appropriate treatment. Some common factors contributing to snoring include:

Anatomy: Certain physical attributes, such as a narrow throat, elongated uvula, or large tonsils, can increase the likelihood of snoring.

Age and Gender: Snoring becomes more prevalent as we age. Men are also more prone to snoring than women, although women can also experience snoring.

Obesity: Excess weight and fatty tissues around the throat can obstruct the airway, leading to snoring.

Alcohol and Sedatives: The consumption of alcohol and sedatives relaxes the throat muscles, contributing to snoring.

Smoking: Smoking irritates the airways and causes inflammation, increasing the chances of snoring.

Nasal Issues: Chronic nasal congestion, deviated septum, or sinus problems can restrict airflow and result in snoring.

Effects of Snoring:

Snoring not only disrupts the quality of sleep for the snorer but can also affect the sleep of their partner. The effects of snoring include:

Sleep Disruption: Snoring often leads to fragmented sleep, resulting in daytime fatigue, irritability, and poor concentration.

Relationship Strain: The loud and persistent snoring noises can strain relationships, causing resentment, frustration, and even separate sleeping arrangements.

Health Risks: Snoring can be a sign of an underlying sleep disorder called sleep apnea, where breathing repeatedly stops and starts during sleep. Sleep apnea is associated with an increased risk of heart disease, stroke, high blood pressure, and other health issues.

Treatment Options:

Thankfully, there are several treatment options available for snoring, ranging from lifestyle changes to medical interventions. The choice of treatment depends on the underlying cause and severity of snoring. Here are some commonly used approaches:

Lifestyle Modifications:

Weight Loss: Shedding excess weight can reduce the fatty tissues around the throat and improve airflow.
Sleeping Position: Elevating the head or sleeping on the side instead of the back can alleviate snoring.

Avoiding Alcohol and Sedatives: Limiting the consumption of alcohol and sedatives can help prevent muscle relaxation in the throat.
Nasal Devices:

Nasal Strips: These adhesive strips widen the nostrils, improving nasal airflow and reducing snoring.
Nasal Dilators: These devices inserted into the nostrils help keep the air passages open during sleep.
Oral Appliances:

Mandibular Advancement Devices (MADs): These custom-fitted devices resemble mouthguards and help keep the jaw and tongue forward, preventing airway obstruction.
Continuous Positive Airway Pressure (CPAP):

CPAP machines deliver a constant stream of air pressure through a mask worn over the nose or nose and mouth. This prevents airway collapse during sleep and is highly effective for sleep apnea-related snoring.

Surgery:
Uvulopalatopharyngoplasty (UPPP):
This surgical procedure removes excess tissues in the throat to widen the airway.
Palatal Implants: Small implants are inserted into the soft palate
to stiffen it and reduce snoring vibrations.

Septoplasty: This surgery corrects a deviated septum, improving nasal airflow and reducing snoring.
Tonsillectomy and Adenoidectomy: Removal of the tonsils and adenoids can be beneficial if they are causing airway obstruction and snoring.
It is important to consult a healthcare professional to determine the most suitable treatment option based on individual circumstances and medical history.

Snoring Prevention:

In addition to treatment options, adopting certain preventive measures can help reduce the frequency and severity of snoring:

Maintain a Healthy Lifestyle: Regular exercise, a balanced diet, and weight management can reduce the risk of snoring caused by obesity.

Create a Sleep-Friendly Environment: Ensure a comfortable sleep environment, with a supportive mattress, appropriate room temperature, and minimal noise disturbances.

Establish Consistent Sleep Patterns: Maintaining a regular sleep schedule and practicing good sleep hygiene can promote better sleep quality and reduce snoring tendencies.

Allergy Management: If allergies contribute to nasal congestion and snoring, taking appropriate measures such as using air purifiers, avoiding allergens, and using nasal saline rinses can be helpful.

Quit Smoking: Quitting smoking can improve overall respiratory health and reduce the risk of snoring.

Conclusion
Snoring is a common sleep disorder that can significantly impact sleep quality, relationships, and overall well-being. Understanding the causes and effects of snoring is essential in seeking appropriate treatment.

Lifestyle modifications, nasal devices, oral appliances, CPAP therapy, and surgery are among the treatment options available.

Preventive measures such as maintaining a healthy lifestyle, creating a sleep-friendly environment, and managing allergies can also help reduce snoring. If you or your partner experience chronic and disruptive snoring, it is advisable to consult a healthcare professional to assess the underlying causes and determine the most effective treatment approach. With proper management, snoring can be alleviated, leading to improved sleep and overall quality of life.

Facts about Snoring:

Snoring is the sound produced when the flow of air through the mouth and nose is partially obstructed during sleep.
Approximately 45% of adults snore occasionally, while about 25% snore habitually.
Snoring occurs more frequently in men than in women.
Snoring tends to increase with age, as the throat muscles become weaker.

Certain factors, such as obesity, alcohol consumption, smoking, and nasal congestion, can contribute to snoring.
Snoring can disrupt sleep, leading to daytime drowsiness and decreased productivity.

It is estimated that snoring can reach a sound level of up to 90 decibels, which is equivalent to the noise produced by a lawnmower.

Snoring can cause relationship problems and disturbances in the sleep of bed partners.

Sleep apnea, a serious sleep disorder, is characterized by loud snoring, pauses in breathing, and gasping or choking during sleep.

Snoring can be an indicator of an underlying health condition, such as nasal polyps, deviated septum, or obesity.

People who snore are more prone to developing high blood pressure and cardiovascular diseases.

Snoring can lead to chronic headaches, sore throat, and dry mouth upon waking up.

Snoring can be hereditary, meaning that if your parents snore, you are more likely to snore as well.

Snoring can worsen during pregnancy due to hormonal changes, weight gain, and increased blood flow.

Sleeping position can influence snoring, as sleeping on your back may lead to more pronounced snoring.

Tricks to Stop Snoring:

Maintain a healthy weight: Losing excess weight can reduce the fatty tissues in the throat that contribute to snoring.

Avoid alcohol and sedatives: These substances relax the throat muscles, increasing the likelihood of snoring.
Sleep on your side: Sleeping on your side can help keep the airway open and

reduce snoring. You can use a body pillow or place a tennis ball in a sock and pin it to the back of your pajamas to discourage sleeping on your back.

Elevate your head: Sleeping with an elevated head can help open up the nasal passages and reduce snoring. You can use a firm pillow or elevate the head of your bed.

Keep nasal passages clear: Use saline nasal sprays or nasal strips to help keep your nasal passages clear, reducing congestion and snoring.

Avoid smoking: Smoking irritates the tissues in the throat and can lead to nasal congestion, making snoring worse.

Stay hydrated: Drinking plenty of water can help thin the mucus in your throat and reduce snoring.

Practice good sleep hygiene: Establish a regular sleep schedule, create a comfortable sleep environment, and ensure you get enough sleep each night to minimize snoring.

Try throat exercises: Strengthening the muscles in your throat through exercises like singing, playing the didgeridoo, or doing specific throat exercises can help reduce snoring.

Consider using nasal devices: Nasal dilators or nasal strips can help keep your nasal passages open, making it easier to breathe and reducing snoring.

Remember, if snoring persists or is accompanied by other symptoms like excessive daytime sleepiness, gasping for breath during sleep, or pauses in breathing, it is important to consult a healthcare professional for a proper diagnosis and treatment.

Chapter3

The disadvantages of sleeping with a snoring person in the same room

What to do if you are a snoring person before sleeping

What to do if your wife or husband snores at night

The disadvantages of sleeping with a snoring person in the same room

Sleeping with a snoring person in the same room can have several disadvantages, which can affect both the snorer and the person sharing the room. Here are some common drawbacks:

Disrupted Sleep: Snoring can disrupt your sleep patterns and lead to fragmented or poor-quality sleep. The loud and constant noise can wake you up or prevent you from falling asleep altogether, resulting in sleep deprivation.

Fatigue and Daytime Sleepiness: Due to disrupted sleep, both the snorer and the person sharing the room may experience daytime sleepiness, which can affect concentration, mood, and overall productivity.

Health Issues: Chronic snoring can be a symptom of a more significant underlying health condition, such as sleep apnea. Sleep apnea is a potentially serious disorder that causes breathing interruptions during sleep.

Sharing a room with someone who has sleep apnea can increase the risk of various health issues for both individuals, including high blood pressure, heart problems, and cognitive impairments.

Relationship Strain: Constant snoring can strain relationships, especially if the snorer's sleep disturbance consistently affects the sleep quality of their partner. The lack of restful sleep can lead to irritability, frustration, and conflicts between partners.

Sleep Disturbances for Others: Snoring not only affects the person sharing the room but can also disturb others nearby. If you live in a shared living situation or have neighbors close by, the snoring noise may disturb their sleep as well.

Negative Impact on Mental Health: The chronic sleep disruptions caused by snoring can contribute to mental health issues such as anxiety and depression. Sleep deprivation can exacerbate existing mental health conditions or even lead to the development of new ones.

Reduced Productivity: Both the snorer and the person sharing the room may experience reduced productivity and cognitive performance due to insufficient sleep. Concentration, memory, and problem-solving abilities can all be negatively affected.

Reliance on Separate Sleeping

Arrangements: In some cases, the disadvantages of sleeping with a snoring person may lead to the need for separate sleeping arrangements. This can impact the intimacy and closeness of a relationship, as well as logistical challenges if space or separate bedrooms are not readily available.

It's important to note that these disadvantages can vary in severity depending on the volume and frequency of the snoring, the underlying causes, and the individuals involved. If snoring is causing significant issues, it may be beneficial to seek medical advice to address the root cause and explore potential solutions.

What to do if you are a snoring person before sleeping

If you are someone who snores, it's important to address the issue proactively to ensure a restful night's sleep for yourself and your loved ones. In this article, we will explore several practical steps you can take to alleviate snoring before going to bed.

By incorporating these strategies into your nightly routine, you can significantly reduce snoring and enjoy a more peaceful slumber.

Maintain a Healthy Lifestyle:
A healthy lifestyle plays a crucial role in reducing snoring. Excess weight, particularly around the neck and throat area, can contribute to airway blockages, leading to snoring.

Engage in regular physical activity and follow a balanced diet to maintain a healthy weight. Avoid consuming heavy meals, alcohol, and sedatives close to bedtime, as they can relax the throat muscles and exacerbate snoring.

Sleep Position:

The position in which you sleep can influence snoring. Sleeping on your back often leads to the tongue and soft tissues in the throat falling backward, obstructing the airway and causing snoring.

Try sleeping on your side instead, as this can help keep the airway open. You can use pillows or other aids designed to encourage side sleeping and keep you in the correct position throughout the night.

Elevate Your Head:

Elevating your head while sleeping can aid in reducing snoring. Using an extra pillow or a wedge pillow to elevate your head and upper body by a few inches helps to keep the airway open and prevent the tongue from blocking the throat.
Experiment with different pillow configurations to find what works best for you and promotes snore-free sleep.

Nasal Dilators and Strips:

For individuals whose snoring originates from nasal congestion or narrow nasal passages, nasal dilators, and adhesive nasal strips can be effective solutions. Nasal dilators are small devices that are inserted into the nostrils to improve airflow, while nasal strips work by opening the nasal passages externally. Both options can help to reduce snoring by enhancing nasal breathing.

Keep Your Bedroom Air Moist:

Dry air can contribute to snoring, as it irritates the throat and nasal passages. To combat this, consider using a humidifier in your bedroom, especially during dry seasons or in arid climates. The increased moisture in the air can help alleviate congestion and reduce snoring.

Regular Exercise for Throat Muscles:

Just like any other muscle in the body, the throat muscles can benefit from regular exercise.

Performing specific throat exercises, such as singing, playing certain wind instruments, or even simple exercises like swallowing, chewing, and sticking out your tongue, can strengthen the muscles and reduce the likelihood of snoring.

Seek Professional Help:

If your snoring persists despite trying various self-help remedies, it may be advisable to consult a healthcare professional or sleep specialist.
They can evaluate your situation, identify any underlying medical conditions contributing to snoring, and recommend appropriate treatment options.

These may include oral appliances, continuous positive airway pressure (CPAP) machines, or surgical interventions, depending on the severity and cause of your snoring.

Remember that addressing snoring is not only beneficial for your well-being but also for the overall harmony and tranquility of your household. With consistency and patience, you can make significant progress in reducing snoring and achieving a more restful night's sleep.

Lastly, it's important to note that while the strategies mentioned in this article can be effective for many individuals, snoring can sometimes be a symptom of a more serious underlying condition, such as sleep apnea.

If you experience excessive daytime sleepiness, morning headaches, pauses in breathing during sleep, or other concerning symptoms, it is essential to consult a healthcare professional for a comprehensive evaluation.

Prioritize your sleep health and take the necessary steps to address snoring. By doing so, you can enhance your overall well-being, improve the quality of your sleep, and wake up each morning feeling refreshed and ready to tackle the day ahead.

Conclusion:
Snoring can be a disruptive issue that affects both your sleep quality and that of your bed partner. By adopting healthy lifestyle habits, making changes to your sleep position, utilizing aids like nasal dilators and strips, and exploring throat exercises, you can take proactive steps to minimize snoring before going to bed. Additionally, don't hesitate to seek professional guidance if your snoring persists or worsens over time.

By implementing these strategies and seeking appropriate help, you can improve the quality of your sleep and wake up feeling refreshed and energized, while also fostering a more peaceful sleep environment for those around you.

What to do if your wife or husband snores at night

Sleep is essential for our physical and mental well-being. However, when you share a bed with a spouse who snores, it can be a source of frustration, leading to disturbed sleep and potential strain on your relationship.

Snoring is a common issue that affects many people, and it's important to address it in a considerate and understanding manner. If your wife or husband snores at night, here are some practical steps you can take to alleviate the problem and improve both of your sleep quality.

1. Open Communication: Approach the issue with kindness and empathy. Start by having an open and honest conversation with your spouse about their snoring. Express your concern for their health and well-being and how it affects your sleep. Remember to maintain a non-confrontational tone and assure them that finding a solution is a joint effort.

2. Encourage a Healthy Lifestyle: Many cases of snoring can be linked to unhealthy lifestyle habits. Encourage your spouse to maintain a healthy weight, engage in regular exercise, and avoid smoking or excessive alcohol consumption. These lifestyle changes can reduce the severity of snoring and improve overall sleep quality.

3. Sleep Positions: Certain sleeping positions can contribute to snoring. Encourage your spouse to sleep on their side instead of their back. You can provide additional support by placing pillows or rolled-up blankets behind their back to help them maintain the side-sleeping position throughout the night.

4. Elevate the Head: Elevating the head can help open up the airways and reduce snoring. You can achieve this by using an extra pillow or investing in an adjustable bed that allows you to raise the head position. Alternatively, consider using a specially designed wedge pillow that helps to keep the head and neck elevated.

5. Nasal Dilators and Strips: Nasal dilators are small devices that can be inserted into the nostrils to improve airflow. These devices work by widening the nasal passages, reducing congestion, and minimizing snoring. Nasal strips can also be helpful as they work externally by opening up the nasal passages.

6. Humidifiers: Dry air can irritate the airways and contribute to snoring. Using a humidifier in the bedroom can add moisture to the air, reducing congestion and promoting clearer breathing. Opt for a cool mist humidifier for safety and ensure regular cleaning to prevent the growth of mold or bacteria.

7. Earplugs and White Noise: If the snoring continues to disrupt your sleep, consider using earplugs or playing white noise in the background. These can help mask the sound of snoring, allowing you to drift off to sleep more easily.

8. Seek Professional Help: If the snoring persists despite your efforts, it may be necessary to seek professional help. Encourage your spouse to consult with a healthcare provider, who can diagnose any underlying medical conditions contributing to the snoring and provide appropriate treatment options. They may recommend a sleep study or refer your spouse to a specialist, such as an otolaryngologist or a sleep medicine physician.

9. Separate Sleeping Arrangements: In some cases, it may be necessary to consider separate sleeping arrangements temporarily. This can provide both you and your spouse with the opportunity to get a good night's sleep while working on finding a long-term solution. Separate bedrooms or a guest room can be utilized until the snoring issue is resolved.

10. Patience and Support: Dealing with snoring can be frustrating, but it's crucial to approach the issue with patience and support. Remember that your spouse may feel embarrassed or self-conscious about their snoring. Offer reassurance and let them know that you are committed to finding a solution together.

It's important to address snoring as a couple to prevent it from negatively impacting your sleep
and your relationship. By following these steps and maintaining open communication, you can work together to find a solution that allows both of you to enjoy a restful sleep.

11. Explore Anti-Snoring Devices: There are numerous anti-snoring devices available on the market that can help reduce or eliminate snoring. For example, oral appliances can be custom-made by a dentist to keep the airway open during sleep. These devices work by repositioning the jaw or tongue to prevent obstruction. Other options include tongue stabilizing devices or mandibular advancement devices. Research and discuss these options with your spouse to determine which one might be most suitable.

12. Lifestyle Changes: Encourage your spouse to make certain lifestyle changes that can contribute to reducing snoring. These changes include maintaining a consistent sleep schedule, avoiding heavy meals close to bedtime, and managing stress levels. Additionally, they should stay hydrated throughout the day and keep their bedroom environment conducive to sleep by ensuring it's dark, quiet, and cool.

13. Consider Allergies and Nasal Congestion: Allergies and nasal congestion can worsen snoring. If your spouse frequently experiences these issues, they should seek treatment to alleviate the symptoms. This may involve avoiding triggers, using nasal sprays or antihistamines, or consulting an allergist for further evaluation and treatment options.

14. Continuous Positive Airway Pressure (CPAP): If your spouse has been diagnosed with obstructive sleep apnea, a condition characterized by pauses in breathing during sleep, a CPAP machine may be recommended. CPAP therapy involves wearing a mask over the nose or mouth that delivers a continuous flow of air, keeping the airway open and preventing snoring. Encourage your spouse to comply with their prescribed treatment and provide support in adjusting to the therapy.

15. Sleep Study: In some cases, a sleep study may be necessary to determine the underlying cause of snoring. A sleep study, conducted in a sleep clinic or at home with specialized equipment, monitors various aspects of sleep, including breathing patterns, oxygen levels, and brain activity. The results can help identify any sleep disorders or abnormalities that contribute to snoring, guiding appropriate treatment recommendations.

16. Maintain a Sleep-Friendly Environment: Create a sleep-friendly environment that promotes relaxation and quality sleep. Keep the bedroom clean, clutter-free, and well-ventilated. Invest in a comfortable mattress and pillows that provide adequate support. Use blackout curtains or an eye mask to block out excess light, and consider using white noise machines or relaxing music to drown out disruptive sounds.

17. Seek Couples Therapy: If snoring continues to cause significant strain on your relationship, seeking couples therapy can be beneficial. A therapist can provide guidance on effective communication strategies, help you navigate any underlying relationship issues, and provide tools to manage the impact of snoring on your emotional connection.

Remember, resolving snoring requires patience, understanding, and a collaborative approach.

By actively working together, you can find effective strategies to minimize snoring and create a peaceful sleeping environment for both you and your spouse. Prioritize your health and the health of your relationship by addressing snoring and its impact on your sleep quality.